THE GALLSTONE-FRIENDLY DIET FOR SENIORS

A Complete Diet Guide to Prevent Gallstone Formation, Support Gallbladder Health, Reduce Discomfort, and Maintain a Healthy Weight

DR LANA BROWN, RN

Copyright Page

© 2024 by Dr. Lana Brown.

All rights reserved. No part of this cookbook may be reproduced, distributed, or transmitted in any form or by any means, including photocopying, recording, or other electronic or mechanical methods, without the prior written permission of the author, except in the case of brief quotations embodied in critical reviews and certain other noncommercial uses permitted by copyright law.

For permissions requests, write to the author at www.thelanabrown.com

Table of Contents

Copyright Page 2

Table of Contents 3

INTRODUCTION 1

UNDERSTANDING GALLSTONES 5

    Causes and Risk Factors 7

    Recognizing Warning Signs 8

    The Impact of Gallstones on Seniors 9

WHY SENIORS ARE PRONE TO GALLSTONES .. 11

    Age-Related Changes in the Body 13

    Common Health Issues in Seniors 13

    The Role of Medications 14

    Lifestyle Factors 15

THE IMPORTANCE OF DIET IN MANAGING GALLSTONES 17

    How Diet Affects Gallstones 18

Overview of a Gallstone-Friendly Diet 19

Common Supplements for Gallstone Prevention 21

GETTING STARTED ON THE GALLSTONE DIET 24

Understanding Nutritional Needs for Seniors . 24

Identifying Problematic Foods 26

Foods to Include and Avoid 27

GALLSTONE-FRIENDLY BREAKFAST RECIPES FOR SENIORS 32

Smoked Salmon Breakfast Wraps 32

Blueberry Almond Chia Pudding 34

Fig & Ricotta Overnight Oats 35

Spinach-Avocado Smoothie 36

Cinnamon Streusel Rolls 37

Peanut Butter & Chia Berry Jam English Muffin 41

Creamy Blueberry-Pecan Oatmeal.................... 42

Raspberry Yogurt Cereal Bowl 44

Rhubarb Oat Muffins... 45

Apple Cinnamon Chia Pudding 48

GALLSTONE-FRIENDLY LUNCH RECIPES FOR SENIORS 51

Sheet-Pan Chicken with Peaches and Tomatoes 51

Healthy Pancakes... 54

Red Chilli & Bean Soup...................................... 56

Gnocchi with a Tomato and Basil Sauce 58

Red Super Soup 61

Beef and Broccoli 63

Bahn Mi Noodle Bowl.. 66

Spiced Tofu Scramble 68

California Walnut and Roasted Carrot Hummus 70

Baked Stuffed Chickpea Cutlets 72

GALLSTONE-FRIENDLY DINNER RECIPES FOR SENIORS 75

Seared Tuna with Bulgur & Chickpea Salad 75

Delicious Chickpea Tuna Salad 78

Spaghetti Squash with Roasted Tomatoes, Beans & Almond Pesto 80

Classic Tuna Niçoise Salad 83

Butternut Squash & Black Bean Enchiladas 87

Red Lentil Soup with Saffron 89

Lemon-Herb Salmon with Caponata & Farro .. 92

Tomatoes with Garlic & Olives 95

White Bean Soup with Pasta 96

Spanish Omelette 99

Lentil Stew with Salsa Verde 101

Black Bean Wraps with Greens 103

Chopped Veggie Grain Bowls with Turmeric Dressing 106

GALLSTONE-FRIENDLY APPETIZER RECIPES FOR SENIORS 108

Homemade Salsa 108

Tomatillo Salsa Verde 109

Puerto Rican Tostones 111

Classic Chili Lime Crispy Chickpeas 113

Sriracha Buffalo Cauliflower Bites 115

Savory Crispy Chicken Strips And Veggies 117

Summer Cauliflower Salad 120

GALLSTONE-FRIENDLY SALAD RECIPES FOR SENIORS 124

Pesto Pasta Salad 124

Picnic Salad with Vegetarian Chicken Style Pieces 127

Winter California Walnut Slaw 130

Super Christmas Salad 131

Loch Duart Salmon Nicoise with Charred Lemon Dressing 133

Salmon with Potato Salad and Horseradish Yogurt 137

Coleslaw - 100% plant-based! 140

Dukkah-crusted halloumi salad 142

For the dressing 143

Mackerel with Red Pepper Quinoa Salad 145

Tuna Beetroot Avocado and Walnut Salad 147

Mango salad with Quorn Fillets 149

BBQ Teriyaki Fillets and Pineapple Buddha Bowl
.... 151

THE ROLE OF NUTRITION IN PREVENTION AND MANAGEMENT OF GALLSTONE 157

INTRODUCTION

Gallstones are deposits of solidified substances found in bile, such as cholesterol. They are common and may not always produce symptoms. Your gallbladder, a small organ located in your upper right abdomen just below your liver, stores bile—a green-yellow liquid that aids digestion. Issues with your gallbladder typically arise when something, like a gallstone, blocks its bile duct.

Most gallstones are formed when substances found in bile, like cholesterol, harden. Although they are quite common, they are often asymptomatic. However, about 10 percent of people diagnosed with gallstones will develop noticeable symptoms within five years.

Symptoms of gallstones can include pain in the upper right abdomen or the center of your stomach, especially after eating fatty foods, like fried items. This pain, often called gallbladder pain, can occur at almost any time but usually lasts only a few hours, though it can feel severe.

If gallstones are left untreated or undiagnosed, symptoms may escalate to include a high temperature, rapid heartbeat, jaundice (yellowing of the skin and eyes), itchy skin, diarrhea, chills, confusion, and loss of appetite. These symptoms can indicate a gallbladder infection or inflammation of the gallbladder, liver, or pancreas. Because the symptoms of gallstones can mimic those of other serious conditions, such as appendicitis and pancreatitis, it is crucial to seek medical attention if you experience any of these issues.

Most of the time, treatment for gallstones is unnecessary unless they cause pain. You might pass gallstones without even noticing. However, if you are in pain, your doctor will likely recommend surgery. In rare cases, medication may be used. For those at high risk of surgery complications, there are a few nonsurgical treatments available. However, these treatments do not guarantee that gallstones will not return, meaning you may need to monitor your condition for a long time.

While there is no guaranteed way to prevent gallstones, cholesterol plays a significant role in their formation. If you have a family history of gallstones, your doctor may suggest limiting foods high in saturated fat.

CHAPTER I

UNDERSTANDING GALLSTONES

Gallstones are small, solid lumps that form in bile, a digestive liquid produced by the liver and stored in the gallbladder. The gallbladder, a pear-shaped pouch about 9 cm long and 4.5 cm wide when full, plays a vital role in digestion by storing bile between meals. When we eat, the gallbladder releases bile through the cystic duct into the main bile duct, which then delivers it to the small bowel. Bile is essential for digesting and absorbing fats from food. However, in some people, bile can solidify and form gallstones, which can lead to various health issues.

Gallstones affect approximately 10 to 15 percent of the population, with a higher incidence in women compared to men. They are particularly common in females who have an unhealthy body weight and have had children. Recently, the prevalence of gallstones has been rising among younger females and teenagers, which is thought to be related to changes in dietary patterns. For seniors, the likelihood of developing symptoms from gallstones increases with age. By the time individuals reach 60, nearly a quarter of females and a smaller proportion of males may experience symptoms related to gallstones.

For seniors, the impact of gallstones can be significant, as the risk of experiencing symptoms and complications grows with age. Regular monitoring and a proactive approach to managing gallstones are crucial for maintaining the health and quality of life for older adults. While specific dietary tips are not provided here, it's important for healthcare providers to consider the overall health status and nutritional needs of seniors to manage gallstones effectively and prevent related complications.

Causes and Risk Factors

Gallstones form when bile, a digestive liquid produced by the liver and stored in the gallbladder, becomes imbalanced. Cholesterol stones are the most common type and are believed to form when bile contains too much cholesterol, too much bilirubin, not enough bile salts, or when the gallbladder does not empty properly. In contrast, pigment stones tend to develop in people with conditions like cirrhosis, biliary tract infections, or hereditary blood disorders such as sickle cell anemia. The exact causes of pigment stones remain uncertain. For seniors, the risk of developing gallstones increases with age, and factors such as obesity, hormonal changes, and a sedentary lifestyle can exacerbate this risk.

Recognizing Warning Signs

Initially, gallstones may not cause any symptoms, which are referred to as "silent stones." However, as gallstones grow larger or obstruct bile ducts, they can lead to painful attacks. Common symptoms include steady, severe pain in the upper abdomen that can last from 30 minutes to several hours, pain between the shoulder blades or in the right shoulder, nausea, vomiting, fever, chills, and jaundice (yellowing of the skin or eyes). Abdominal bloating, intolerance of fatty foods, belching, and indigestion are also possible signs. Seniors should be particularly vigilant for these symptoms, as they may signal the need for medical attention.

The Impact of Gallstones on Seniors

For seniors, the impact of gallstones can be particularly significant due to the increased likelihood of experiencing symptoms and complications with age. Biliary colic, which occurs when a gallstone temporarily blocks the bile duct and then moves away, serves as a warning sign that should not be ignored. This pain may subside, but it indicates that further issues could arise. If a gallstone causes a blockage and remains stuck, it could lead to more severe complications requiring emergency care. The risk of gallstones causing blockages and persistent symptoms makes it essential for seniors to recognize these signs early and seek appropriate medical advice to manage their condition effectively.

CHAPTER II

WHY SENIORS ARE PRONE TO GALLSTONES

Age is a major risk factor for the formation of gallstones, or cholelithiasis. While it is unclear as to the reasons for this increased prevalence, 38% of women and 22% of men have gallstones by age 90. More than half the cases (50% to 70%) of acute cholecystitis, defined as inflammation, and possibly infection, of the gallbladder, occur in seniors. Ethnicity and race also play a role. Highly prevalent in the geriatric population, acute cholecystitis may occur in the presence or absence of gallstones, although it is almost always due to gallstones. Its severity varies from mild edema to severe inflammation, and even to necrosis or perforation of the gallbladder at its most catastrophic.

Seniors are particularly susceptible to gallstones due to a combination of biological and lifestyle factors. As people age, the risk of gallstone formation increases significantly. By age 90, a substantial percentage of both men and women will have developed gallstones. This heightened prevalence is likely due to age-related changes in the body that affect the composition of bile and the functioning of the gallbladder. Additionally, genetic predisposition and hormonal changes, especially in postmenopausal women, contribute to the higher incidence of gallstones in the elderly population.

Age-Related Changes in the Body

With advancing age, the body's metabolic processes slow down, and the composition of bile may change, leading to an increased likelihood of cholesterol stones. The gallbladder's ability to contract and empty bile efficiently may also diminish, causing bile to become concentrated and facilitating stone formation. These physiological changes make seniors more vulnerable to developing gallstones and experiencing related complications such as acute cholecystitis, where the gallbladder becomes inflamed and possibly infected.

Common Health Issues in Seniors

Seniors often face a range of health issues that can indirectly increase the risk of gallstones. Conditions such as obesity, diabetes, and metabolic syndrome are common in older adults and are known risk factors for gallstone formation. Furthermore, a sedentary lifestyle and dietary habits that include high-fat, high-cholesterol foods can exacerbate the risk. Chronic illnesses that require long-term medication use can also influence bile composition and gallbladder function, further increasing the likelihood of gallstone development.

The Role of Medications

Many seniors take medications for chronic conditions, and some of these medications can affect bile production and gallbladder function. For instance, cholesterol-lowering drugs can alter bile composition, making it more prone to forming stones. Hormone replacement therapy, commonly used by postmenopausal women, can also increase the risk of gallstones. It is important for healthcare providers to monitor the medication regimens of seniors and consider the potential impact on gallbladder health.

Lifestyle Factors

Lifestyle factors play a crucial role in the development and management of gallstones in seniors. A hypercaloric diet rich in carbohydrates and poor in fiber, combined with obesity, is a significant risk factor for gallstone formation. However, adopting a healthy lifestyle can mitigate this risk. Regular exercise, an appropriate diet low in saturated fats and high in fiber, and maintaining a healthy body weight are decisive preventive measures. Seniors should be encouraged to stay active and make dietary choices that support overall digestive health to reduce the likelihood of gallstone complications.

The increased prevalence of gallstones in seniors is a multifaceted issue influenced by age-related physiological changes, common health issues, medication use, and lifestyle factors. Understanding these factors and implementing preventive measures can help manage the risk and impact of gallstones in the elderly population.

CHAPTER III

THE IMPORTANCE OF DIET IN MANAGING GALLSTONES

A diet rich in nutrient-dense foods like vegetables and fruit may help prevent gallstones. Other foods, including those high in refined sugar and saturated fat, may increase your risk.

Gallstones, small stones usually made up of bile, form in the gallbladder and can cause significant discomfort and health issues. Diet plays a crucial role in managing and preventing gallstones, especially for seniors. A well-balanced diet can prevent the formation of gallstones and reduce the likelihood of symptoms or complications.

How Diet Affects Gallstones

The gallbladder stores bile produced by the liver and releases it into the small intestine to help digest food. Eating a diet rich in fried and fatty foods may increase your risk of developing gallstones, which can subsequently increase your risk of gallbladder disease, such as porcelain gallbladder and cancer.

On the other hand, a diet high in fiber, low in unhealthy fats, and rich in fruits, vegetables, and whole grains can support gallbladder health. Such a diet helps maintain a healthy weight, regulate cholesterol levels, and ensure proper digestion, all of which are vital in preventing gallstone formation.

Overview of a Gallstone-Friendly Diet

- Fruits, Vegetables, and Whole Grains: A diet rich in fruits, vegetables, and whole grains is beneficial for gallbladder health. These foods are high in fiber, which supports digestion and helps prevent gallstones. Cruciferous vegetables, berries, citrus fruits, legumes, and whole grains like brown rice, quinoa, and oats are particularly recommended.
- Healthy Fats: Choosing healthy fats over unhealthy fats is crucial. Healthy fats, such as those found in nuts, peanuts, olive oil, and omega-3 fatty acids from fish or fish oil supplements, can help regulate gallbladder contractions and improve bile quality.

- Plant-Based Proteins: Incorporating plant-based proteins like beans, nuts, lentils, soy products, and plant-based meat alternatives can also help prevent gallbladder conditions.
- Regular Coffee Consumption: Studies have shown that regular coffee consumption can reduce the risk of symptomatic gallstones. Drinking one to six cups of coffee daily may help lower the risk.
- Moderate Alcohol Consumption: Moderate alcohol intake has been linked to a decreased risk of gallstones. However, it is important to consume alcohol in moderation to avoid other health risks.
- Regular and Frequent Mealtimes: Eating meals on a regular schedule and avoiding long gaps between meals can help prevent gallstones. Regular fasting for more than 16

to 18 hours per day may increase the risk of gallstones.

Common Supplements for Gallstone Prevention

Certain dietary supplements, including vitamins, minerals, and herbs, may prove beneficial for gallbladder disease. However, no supplement will completely heal your gallbladder on its own. Supplements should only complement other treatment options for any health condition, including gallbladder disease.

- Magnesium: Some studies suggest that magnesium supplements may reduce the risk of gallstones and other gallbladder issues. However, more research is needed to confirm these findings.

- Dandelion: Dandelion root is believed to increase bile flow and may help prevent gallstones, although solid scientific evidence is lacking.
- Vitamin C: As an antioxidant, vitamin C may protect against gallstones. Some studies have found that regular vitamin C consumption is associated with lower rates of gallstones.
- Vitamin E: This fat-soluble vitamin and antioxidant may protect against gallstones. Higher vitamin E levels have been linked to a lower risk of gallstone disease.
- Milk Thistle: Milk thistle has been used for centuries as a natural treatment for gallstones. However, more research is needed to determine its effectiveness.

Maintaining a healthy diet is essential for managing and preventing gallstones, especially in seniors. A diet rich in fiber, healthy fats, plant-based proteins, and regular coffee consumption, along with moderate alcohol intake and regular meal schedules, can support gallbladder health. Additionally, certain supplements may offer benefits, although they should be used in conjunction with other treatment options.

CHAPTER IV

GETTING STARTED ON THE GALLSTONE DIET

Maintaining a healthy diet is universally important, but it becomes increasingly significant as we age. After 65, seniors may face unique dietary challenges due to age-related metabolic changes and lifestyle adjustments.

Understanding Nutritional Needs for Seniors

The gallbladder, a small organ that stores bile, plays a role in digesting fats. Although not essential for survival, a healthy gallbladder is important for digestive health. Gallstones can form when bile becomes imbalanced, leading to symptoms like abdominal pain and nausea. While diet alone cannot cure gallstones, it can help prevent their formation and alleviate symptoms.

Risk Factors for Gallstones:

- Gender and Weight: Women are at higher risk than men, and obesity or rapid weight loss increases the likelihood of gallstone formation.
- Dietary Influence: Diets high in fat and cholesterol but low in fiber contribute to gallstone development. A balanced diet that supports gallbladder health is crucial for prevention.

Identifying Problematic Foods

Proper nutrition is essential for maintaining critical functions like heart health, kidney function, and bone regeneration. Therefore, a focus on nutrient-rich foods and balanced meals is crucial to support these systems and promote overall well-being.

Health Risks Associated with Poor Diet:

- Malnutrition and Weight Fluctuations: Seniors are at risk of malnutrition due to factors like decreased appetite, difficulty chewing, or medical conditions affecting nutrient absorption. Weight changes, whether due to unintentional weight loss or gain, can lead to complications such as osteoporosis and vitamin deficiencies.

- Lifestyle Factors: Life changes such as the loss of a spouse or diminished independence can impact a senior's willingness or ability to maintain a healthy diet. Emotional and social factors can also play a role, influencing dietary habits and overall health.

Foods to Include and Avoid

Healthy Foods for Gallbladder Health:

Eating a diet that supports gallbladder function involves incorporating foods that are low in fat and high in fiber:

Fresh Fruits and Vegetables: High in essential vitamins and fiber, fruits and vegetables support overall health. Citrus fruits, bell peppers, leafy greens, and tomatoes are particularly beneficial.

Whole Grains: Foods like whole-wheat bread, brown rice, oats, and bran cereal provide necessary fiber and help maintain digestive health.

Lean Proteins: Opt for poultry, fish, beans, tofu, and nuts instead of red meats and high-fat dairy products.

Low-Fat Dairy: Choose low-fat options such as skim milk or low-fat cheese, or consider milk alternatives like almond or oat milk.

Foods to Avoid:

To prevent gallstone symptoms and complications, limit the intake of:

High-Fat Foods: Avoid fried foods, highly processed snacks, whole-milk dairy products, and fatty cuts of meat.

Refined Carbohydrates: Foods high in refined sugars and fats can exacerbate gallbladder issues.

Tips for Dietary Adjustments:

- Gradual Weight Loss: If overweight, aim for a slow and steady weight loss of 1-2 pounds per week to avoid rapid changes that may trigger gallstones.
- Regular Meals: Eat regular, balanced meals and avoid skipping breakfast to maintain healthy bile production and gallbladder function.
- Cooking Methods: Use cooking methods that reduce fat, such as steaming, boiling, or grilling instead of frying.

Special Considerations for Older Adults

- Older adults often face unique challenges when it comes to nutrition. Despite having lower calorie needs, nutrient requirements remain high due to changes in metabolism and health conditions. Focus on:
- Protein Intake: Ensure adequate protein consumption from sources like seafood, dairy, and plant-based alternatives to maintain muscle mass and overall health.
- Vitamin B12: With age, absorption of vitamin B12 can decline. Incorporate fortified foods or discuss supplements with a healthcare provider to meet daily needs.
- Diet Quality: Improve diet quality by increasing intake of fruits, vegetables, whole grains, and dairy while reducing added sugars, saturated fats, and sodium.

CHAPTER V

GALLSTONE-FRIENDLY BREAKFAST RECIPES FOR SENIORS

Smoked Salmon Breakfast Wraps

INGREDIENTS

⅓ cup light cream cheese spread

1 tablespoon snipped fresh chives

1 teaspoon finely shredded lemon peel

1 tablespoon lemon juice

4 6 to 7-inch whole wheat flour tortillas

3 ounces thinly sliced, smoked salmon (lox-style), cut into strips

1 small zucchini, trimmed

4 Lemon wedges

INSTRUCTIONS

In a small bowl, stir together cream cheese, chives, lemon peel, and lemon juice until smooth. Spread evenly over tortillas, leaving a 1/2-inch border around the edges.

Divide salmon among tortillas, placing it on the bottom half of each tortilla. To make zucchini ribbons, draw a sharp vegetable peeler lengthwise along the zucchini to cut very thin slices. Place zucchini ribbons on top of salmon. Starting from the bottom, roll up tortillas. Cut in half. If desired, serve with lemon wedges.

Blueberry Almond Chia Pudding

INGREDIENTS

½ cup unsweetened almond milk or other nondairy milk beverage

2 tablespoons chia seeds

2 teaspoons pure maple syrup

⅛ teaspoon almond extract

½ cup fresh blueberries, divided

1 tablespoon toasted slivered almonds, divided

INSTRUCTIONS

Stir together almond milk (or other nondairy milk beverage), chia, maple syrup and almond extract in a small bowl. Cover and refrigerate for at least 8 hours and up to 3 days.

When ready to serve, stir the pudding well. Spoon about half the pudding into a serving glass (or bowl) and top with half the blueberries and almonds. Add the rest of the pudding and top with the remaining blueberries and almonds.

Fig & Ricotta Overnight Oats

INGREDIENTS

½ cup old-fashioned rolled oats (see Tip)

½ cup water

Pinch of salt

2 tablespoons part-skim ricotta cheese

2 tablespoons chopped dried figs

1 tablespoon toasted sliced almonds

2 teaspoons honey

INSTRUCTIONS

Combine oats, water and salt in a jar or bowl and stir. Cover and refrigerate overnight.

In the morning, heat the oats, if desired, or eat cold. Top with ricotta, figs, almonds and honey.

Spinach-Avocado Smoothie

INGREDIENTS

1 cup nonfat plain yogurt

1 cup fresh spinach

1 frozen banana

¼ avocado

2 tablespoons water

1 teaspoon honey

INSTRUCTIONS

Combine yogurt, spinach, banana, avocado, water and honey in a blender. Puree until smooth.

Cinnamon Streusel Rolls

INGREDIENTS

1 cup fat-free milk plus 2 to 3 teaspoons, divided

2 teaspoons packed brown sugar (see Tip)

¼ cup tub-style 60-70% vegetable oil spread, divided

1 teaspoon salt

¼ cup warm water (110 to 115 degrees F)

1 package active dry yeast

¼ cup refrigerated or frozen egg product, thawed, or 1 egg, lightly beaten

4-4 1/2 cups all-purpose flour (see Tip)

½ cup rolled oats, toasted (see Tip)

2 teaspoons ground cinnamon

¼ cup chopped pecans, toasted (see Tip)

⅓ cup light sour cream

¼ cup powdered sugar

¼ teaspoon vanilla extract

INSTRUCTIONS

Heat and stir 1 cup milk, the brown sugar, 2 tablespoons vegetable oil spread, and the salt in a small saucepan just until warm (110 to 115 degrees F); set aside. Combine the warm water and yeast in a large bowl; let stand for 10 minutes. Add egg and the milk mixture to the yeast mixture. Stir in the flour substitute (if using; see Tip) and as much of the remaining all-purpose flour as you can with a wooden spoon.

Turn out dough onto a lightly floured surface. Knead in enough of the remaining flour to make a moderately soft dough that is smooth and elastic (3 to 5 minutes total). Shape the dough into a ball. Place in a lightly greased bowl, turning once to grease the surface. Cover and let rise in a warm place until double in size (about 1 hour). Punch down the dough. Turn out onto a lightly floured surface. Cover; let rest for 10 minutes.

Meanwhile, lightly grease a 13x9-inch baking pan; set aside. Combine oats and cinnamon in a medium bowl. Using your fingers, blend in the remaining 2 tablespoons vegetable oil spread until the mixture is crumbly. Stir in pecans.

Roll the dough into a 15x8-inch rectangle. Sprinkle with the pecan mixture, leaving a 1-inch space along one of the long sides. Starting from the long side with topping, roll up into a spiral. Pinch the dough to seal seam; slice into 15 equal pieces. Arrange the pieces, cut sides up, in the prepared baking pan. Cover and let rise in a warm place until nearly double in size (about 30 minutes).

Preheat oven to 375 degrees F. Bake for 25 to 30 minutes or until golden. Cool in the pan on a wire rack for 5 minutes.

Meanwhile, combine sour cream, powdered sugar, vanilla, and enough of the remaining 2 to 3 teaspoons milk to make drizzling consistency. Remove the rolls from the pan. Drizzle with icing. Serve warm.

Peanut Butter & Chia Berry Jam English Muffin

INGREDIENTS

½ cup unsweetened mixed frozen berries

2 teaspoons chia seeds

2 teaspoons natural peanut butter

1 whole-wheat English muffin, toasted

INSTRUCTIONS

Microwave berries in a medium microwave-safe bowl for 30 seconds; stir and microwave 30 seconds more. Stir in chia seeds.

Spread peanut butter on the English muffin. Top with the berry-chia mixture.

Creamy Blueberry-Pecan Oatmeal

INGREDIENTS

1 cup water

Pinch of salt

½ cup old-fashioned rolled oats

½ cup blueberries, fresh or frozen, thawed

2 tablespoons nonfat plain Greek yogurt

1 tablespoon toasted chopped pecans

2 teaspoons pure maple syrup

INSTRUCTIONS

Bring water and salt to a boil in a small saucepan. Stir in oats, reduce heat to medium and cook, stirring occasionally, until most of the liquid is absorbed, about 5 minutes. Remove from heat, cover and let stand 2 to 3 minutes. Top with blueberries, yogurt, pecans and syrup.

Tips

Overnight oats variation: Combine 1/2 cup old-fashioned rolled oats with 1/2 cup water and a pinch of salt in a jar or bowl. Cover and refrigerate overnight. In the morning, add toppings. Eat cold or heat up. Makes about 1 cup.

Steel-cut oats variation: Bring 1 cup water and a pinch of salt to a boil in a small saucepan. Add 1/3 cup steel-cut oats, reduce heat to a bare simmer, cover and cook, stirring occasionally, until most of the liquid is absorbed, 15 to 20 minutes. Remove from heat and let stand, covered, 2 to 3 minutes. Add toppings. Makes about 1 cup.

People with celiac disease or gluten-sensitivity should use oats that are labeled "gluten-free," as oats are often cross-contaminated with wheat and barley.

Raspberry Yogurt Cereal Bowl

INGREDIENTS

1 cup nonfat plain yogurt

½ cup mini shredded-wheat cereal

¼ cup fresh raspberries

2 teaspoons mini chocolate chips

1 teaspoon pumpkin seeds

¼ teaspoon ground cinnamon

INSTRUCTIONS

Place yogurt in a bowl and top with shredded wheat, raspberries, chocolate chips, pumpkin seeds and cinnamon.

Rhubarb Oat Muffins

INGREDIENTS

Nonstick cooking spray

1 ¾ cups regular rolled oats

¾ cup whole-wheat pastry flour or whole-wheat flour

½ cup all-purpose flour

½ cup packed brown sugar (see Tip)

1 teaspoon baking powder

½ teaspoon baking soda

¼ teaspoon salt

¾ cup buttermilk

½ cup refrigerated or frozen egg product, thawed, or 2 eggs, lightly beaten

2 tablespoons canola oil

1 teaspoon vanilla

1 cup finely chopped rhubarb

1 tablespoon packed brown sugar (see Tip)

½ teaspoon ground cinnamon

¼ cup chopped walnuts

INSTRUCTIONS

Preheat oven to 350 degrees F. Line twelve 2 1/2-inch muffin cups with paper bake cups; coat paper cups with cooking spray. Or coat muffin cups with cooking spray.

Place 3/4 cup of the oats in a food processor; cover and process until ground. Transfer to a large bowl. Stir in another 3/4 cup of the oats, whole-wheat flour, all-purpose flour, brown sugar, baking powder, baking soda and salt. Make a well in center of flour mixture.

In a medium bowl combine buttermilk, eggs, oil and vanilla. Stir in rhubarb. Add rhubarb mixture all at once to flour mixture; stir just until moistened (batter should be slightly lumpy). Spoon into prepared muffin cups, filling each about three-fourths full.

For streusel topping, in a small bowl stir together brown sugar and cinnamon. Stir in the remaining 1/4 cup oats and walnuts. Sprinkle over batter in muffin cups.

Bake 20 to 22 minutes or until a toothpick comes out clean. Cool in muffin cups on a wire rack for 5 minutes. Remove from muffin cups. Serve warm.

Tips

Tips: If using a sugar substitute for the muffins, we recommend Splenda(R) Brown Sugar Blend. Follow package directions to use 1/2 cup equivalent. Nutrition Per Serving with Substitute: Same as below, except 166 cal, 25 g carb. (6 g sugars).

Apple Cinnamon Chia Pudding

INGREDIENTS

½ cup unsweetened almond milk or other nondairy milk

2 tablespoons chia seeds

2 teaspoons pure maple syrup

¼ teaspoon vanilla extract

¼ teaspoon ground cinnamon

½ cup diced apple, divided

1 tablespoon chopped toasted pecans, divided

INSTRUCTIONS

Stir almond milk (or other nondairy milk), chia, maple syrup, vanilla and cinnamon together in a small bowl. Cover and refrigerate for at least 8 hours and up to 3 days.

When ready to serve, stir well. Spoon about half the pudding into a serving glass (or bowl) and top with half the apple and pecans. Add the rest of the pudding and top with the remaining apple and pecans.

Tips

To make ahead: Refrigerate pudding (Step 1) for up to 3 days. Finish with Step 2 just before serving.

CHAPTER VI

GALLSTONE-FRIENDLY LUNCH RECIPES FOR SENIORS

Sheet-Pan Chicken with Peaches and Tomatoes

INGREDIENTS

1 pound on-vine small tomatoes or cherry tomatoes

1 pound peaches, cut into wedges

1 large red onion, cut into thin half-moons (2 1/2 cups)

4 tablespoon olive oil

Kosher salt

2 cloves garlic, minced

3 tablespoon Dijon-style mustard

2 tablespoon red wine vinegar

2 tablespoon honey

½ teaspoon freshly ground black pepper

8 8 ounce skinless, boneless chicken breast halves

INSTRUCTIONS

Preheat oven to 450°F. Arrange tomatoes, peaches, and onion in a shallow baking pan. Drizzle with 2 Tbsp. oil; sprinkle with 1/2 tsp. salt. Toss to coat; spread in an even layer.

In a large bowl combine remaining 2 Tbsp. oil, the garlic, mustard, vinegar, honey, 1/2 tsp. salt, and 1/2 tsp. freshly ground black pepper. Whisk to combine. Add chicken; turn to coat.*

Arrange chicken breasts in another shallow baking pan. Drizzle chicken with any remaining mustard mixture. Place both pans in oven on separate racks. Roast 20 to 25 minutes or until chicken is done (165°F), stirring tomato mixture halfway and rotating pans top to bottom. Transfer chicken to a cutting board. Let rest 10 minutes. Meanwhile, continue roasting tomato mixture until vegetables just begin to brown.

Cut chicken into thick slices; transfer to a platter and top with tomato mixture. Serves 8.

Tips

If desired, brown the chicken after coating with mustard mixture. In a 12-inch skillet heat 1 Tbsp. olive oil over medium-high. Add half the chicken. Cook 2 minutes on each side or until browned. Transfer to a shallow baking pan. Repeat with remaining chicken, adding more oil to skillet if needed. Roast as directed in Step 3.

Healthy Pancakes

INGREDIENTS

1 seasoned non-stick frying or pancake pan

2 eggs

100g plain flour

300mls semi skimmed milk

1 tablespoon sunflower oil

Rapeseed oil for frying

INSTRUCTIONS

Beat the eggs together in a mixing bowl.

Add the flour and beat until smooth.

Gradually add the milk until you have a smooth batter. Add the oil and mix.

You can prepare the batter in advance and leave to rest in the fridge or use straight away.

Add a teaspoon of rapeseed oil to the frying pan and heat gently, then wipe it away with kitchen paper to season the pan. Add another teaspoon of oil and heat. Do not allow it to pass its smoke point.

Once the oil is hot, ladle in some of the batter into the pan, and tilt it to form a thin even layer. Return any excess batter to the bowl. Leave to cook for 30 seconds to 1 minute.

After this time use a fish slice to ease the pancake away from the sides – if it is cooked it should come away easily and be a golden brown. If not loose then cook a little longer. Once it is cooked on the bottom, flip the pancake over (or toss it if you are feeling brave) and leave to cook for a further 1-2 minutes.

Repeat the process but take care as the pancakes make cook faster as your pan gets hotter. You may need to turn down the heat a little.

Red Chilli & Bean Soup

INGREDIENTS

1 red pepper

1 medium onion

1 celery stick

1 medium carrot

1 clove garlic

2 tbsp olive oil

½ tsp chilli powder or to taste

400g can tomatoes

2 tbsp tomato puree

700ml vegetable stock made from 2 reduced salt stock cubes

1 can mixed beans , drained and rinsed

25g kale leaves, shredded

INSTRUCTIONS

1. De-seed the pepper. Chop the pepper, celery and carrot and the onion and crush the garlic.

2. Heat the oil in a large pan and add the chopped vegetables, saute for about 5 minutes, taking care not to colour the vegetables.

3. Add the chilli powder and cook for a further minute.

4. Puree the tomatoes with a hand-held blender and add to the pan together with the tomato puree and the vegetable stock. Bring to the boil and simmer for 10 minutes.

5. Drain and rinse the mixed beans and stir into the soup along with the shredded kale leaves. Cook for a few minutes until the beans have warmed through and the kale is wilted. Season with pepper and serve.

Gnocchi with a Tomato and Basil Sauce

INGREDIENTS

For the gnocchi:

1kg floury potatoes

1 egg

300g plain flour

For the sauce:

2 tablespoons olive oil

1 onion

2 cloves of garlic

800g chopped tomatoes

1 teaspoon sugar

1 handful of basil

INSTRUCTIONS

For the gnocchi, place the potatoes in a pan of cold water and bring to the boil until tender. Drain and then allow to cool slightly before mashing. Set aside to cool completely.

In the meantime, for the sauce, heat the oil in a saucepan and cook the onion and garlic until soft. Stir in the tomatoes and sugar, then bring to a simmer and leave for 45 minutes. Stir in the basil and it is ready to serve.

Once the potatoes have cooled, season to taste and stir in the egg and flour to form a dough.

Roll out the gnocchi mixture into four sausage shapes and then cut into small pieces.

Place the gnocchi into a pan of boiling water and simmer until they rise to the top.

Serve the gnocchi immediately with the tomato and basil sauce stirred through.

Red Super Soup

INGREDIENTS

1 tablespoon olive oil

2 small red onions, roughly chopped

2 cloves garlic, crushed

1 stick celery, roughly chopped

1 carrot, roughly chopped

250g red cabbage, finely shredded

50g red pepper, roughly chopped

100g red lentils, precooked in boiling water

2 cans chopped tomatoes, (pureed if you are not going to blend the final soup)

½ litre vegetable stock made from 1.5 cubes of reduced salt stock cubes

1 tbsp balsamic vinegar

Ground black pepper

Flat Leaf Parsley, to garnish (Optional)

INSTRUCTIONS

In a large pan, sweat the onions and the garlic in the olive oil for a few minutes until softened, taking care not to colour the onions.

Add the celery and carrots and continue to stir and cook for a few minutes on a low heat

Add the red cabbage, red pepper, cooked lentils, pureed tomatoes and vegetable stock and simmer until all the vegetables are cooked and tender, about 10 minutes

You can use a hand blender to puree the soup if you prefer or serve it with chunky vegetables in a delicious tomato soup

Add a tablespoon of balsamic vinegar and season with black pepper before serving in warm bowls. Garnish with fresh parsley, if using and serve with thick slices of wholemeal bread.

Beef and Broccoli

INGREDIENTS

2 cup sliced yellow onion

1 ½ - 1 ¾ pound beef flank steak or beef bottom round steak, cut across the grain into 4 to 6 portions

½ cup reduced-sodium beef broth

½ cup reduced-sodium soy sauce

3 tablespoon hoisin sauce

2 tablespoon packed dark brown sugar

1 tablespoon rice wine vinegar or cider vinegar

1 tablespoon grated fresh ginger

5 cloves garlic, minced

3 tablespoon water

1 tablespoon cornstarch

4 cup fresh broccoli florets

Toasted sesame seeds (optional)

INSTRUCTIONS

Slow Cooker:

Place onion and meat in a 3 1/2- to 4-qt. slow cooker. In a small bowl combine broth, soy sauce, hoisin, brown sugar, vinegar, ginger, and garlic; pour over meat mixture. Cover; cook on low 8 to 10 hours. Remove meat, reserving onion and cooking liquid in cooker. Cover meat to keep warm. In a small bowl combine 3 Tbsp. water and the cornstarch. Turn heat setting to high. Stir into cooking liquid. Add broccoli. Cover; cook about 15 minutes more or until cooking liquid is thickened and bubbly and broccoli is crisp-tender. Slice meat thinly across the grain. Stir into broccoli mixture. If desired, top with sesame seeds. Serve over rice noodles or rice. Serves 6.

Pressure Cooker:

Place onion and meat in a 6-qt. electric pressure cooker. In a small bowl combine broth, soy sauce, hoisin, brown sugar, vinegar, ginger, and garlic; pour over meat mixture. Lock lid. Set on high pressure. Cook 15 minutes. Immediately release pressure. Remove meat; cover to keep warm. In a small bowl combine 3 Tbsp. water and the cornstarch. Stir into cooking liquid in cooker. Add broccoli. Using the saute setting, cook and stir until cooking liquid is thickened and bubbly and broccoli is crisp-tender. Slice meat thinly across the grain. Stir into broccoli mixture. If desired, top with sesame seeds. Serve over rice noodles or rice. Serves 6.

Bahn Mi Noodle Bowl

INGREDIENTS

1 tablespoon coconut or olive oil

1 pound pork tenderloin, trimmed and cut into bite-size pieces

¼ teaspoon sea salt

¼ teaspoon black pepper

2 cup vegetable stock

½ cup rice vinegar

1 - 2 teaspoon crushed red pepper

1 tablespoon honey

½ teaspoon grated fresh ginger

12 ounce fresh or frozen spiralized carrots (thawed, if frozen)

¼ cup thinly sliced radishes

¼ cup thinly sliced English cucumber

2 tablespoon snipped fresh cilantro

INSTRUCTIONS

In a large straight-sided skillet heat oil over medium-high. Add pork to skillet; season with salt and black pepper. Cook 5 minutes or until no longer pink and edges are browned. Stir in the next five ingredients (through ginger). Cook and stir just until boiling. Stir in spiaralized carrots. Cook about 2 minutes or until heated through and carrots are tender.

Divide pork mixture among shallow bowls. Top with rad

Spiced Tofu Scramble

INGREDIENTS

250gm plain firm tofu, finely chopped or crumbled

1 onion, finely chopped

½ tsp grated ginger

½ tsp turmeric

½ tsp dry roasted cumin seeds, finely ground

½ green chilli deseeded and chopped

1 tsp rapeseed oil

1 tbsp chopped fresh coriander or chive flowers, to serve

INSTRUCTIONS

Gently cook the onion in the oil, in a non-stick pan, until softened.

Add the ginger, turmeric and chilli and cook for another 2 minutes.

Add the tofu to the pan, mix and cook over a low heat for about 5 minutes stirring regularly.

Add the cumin powder and stir.

Serve sprinkled with fresh herbs, over wholemeal bread or with wholemeal chapatti.

California Walnut and Roasted Carrot Hummus

INGREDIENTS

For the hummus:

200g carrots, cut into sticks

1 tsp cumin seeds

1 tbsp extra virgin olive oil

1 x 400g tin chickpeas, drained

2 tbsp tahini

Juice of 1 lemon

80g California walnuts, toasted

Splash of water

Freshly Ground Black Pepper, to taste

To serve:

A handful of green olives, roughly chopped

2 slices of preserved lemons, thinly sliced

Small bunch coriander, roughly chopped or torn

Additional extra virgin olive oil (optional)

INSTRUCTIONS

Preheat the oven to 180°C.

Place the carrots onto a small roasting tray and sprinkle over the cumin and olive oil. Roast in the oven for 25-30 minutes, or until tinged golden.

Place the roasted carrots, chickpeas, tahini, lemon juice and 50g of the California walnuts into a food processor and blitz until smooth, adding in a splash of water if you need to loosen the mixture a little. Season to taste with pepper.

Spoon the hummus into your chosen container, then top with the olives, preserved lemon slices, coriander and leftover walnuts. Drizzle over some extra olive oil.

Baked Stuffed Chickpea Cutlets

INGREDIENTS

Filling

2 tablespoons cottage cheese

2 tablespoons low fat grated cheese

Cutlets

2 cans chickpeas in water

1 teaspoon ginger and garlic paste

2 tablespoons chopped coriander leaves

1 green chilli, finely chopped

4 tablespoons natural low fat yogurt

1 teaspoon dried mint

½ cup breadcrumbs, wholemeal preferably

3 tomatoes, sliced

INSTRUCTIONS

Mix cottage cheese and grated cheese together and keep aside.

Drain the chickpeas and mash finely.

Add ginger/garlic paste, chopped chilli, coriander, pepper and 2 tablespoons of the yogurt and mix lightly.

Divide the mixture into 12 equal balls.

Stuff each with 1 teaspoon of the filling. Cover the filling to form a flat round cutlet.

Mix 2 tablespoons of the remaining yogurt with mint and spread over the round cutlets. Sprinkle each cutlet with bread crumbs to coat on all sides.

Place on a lightly greased baking tray.

Bake at 180C for 20-25 minutes or until cooked through. Serve garnished with sliced tomatoes.

CHAPTER VII

GALLSTONE-FRIENDLY DINNER RECIPES FOR SENIORS

Seared Tuna with Bulgur & Chickpea Salad

INGREDIENTS

½ cup bulgur

¼ cup extra-virgin olive oil, divided

4 teaspoons grated lemon zest, divided

½ cup lemon juice, divided

½ teaspoon salt, divided

¼ teaspoon ground pepper

1 (15 ounce) can no-salt-added chickpeas

¼ cup chopped fresh Italian parsley

¼ cup chopped fresh mint

1 pound tuna, cut into 4 steaks (see Tip)

1 medium yellow onion, thinly sliced

¼ cup chopped fresh dill

INSTRUCTIONS

Bring a kettle of water to a boil. Place bulgur in a large heatproof bowl. Add boiling water to cover by 2 inches. Let stand for 30 minutes. Drain any excess water.

Mix the bulgur with 2 Tbsp. oil, 2 tsp. lemon zest, 1/4 cup lemon juice, 1/4 tsp. salt, and pepper. Add chickpeas, parsley, and mint; stir to combine. Set aside.

Heat the remaining 2 Tbsp. oil in a large skillet over medium-high heat. Add tuna steaks and sear until lightly browned on one side, 2 to 3 minutes. Flip the tuna and cook until lightly browned on the other side. Transfer to a plate.

Reduce heat to medium. Add onion to the pan and cook, stirring occasionally, until translucent, about 5 minutes. Reduce heat to medium-low. Return the tuna steaks to the pan, cover, and cook, flipping once, until the tuna begins to flake when tested with a fork (it will be slightly pink in the center), 3 to 4 minutes per side.

Meanwhile, combine dill with the remaining 1/4 cup lemon juice and 1/4 tsp. salt in a small bowl.

Transfer the tuna to a serving platter. Spoon the onions over the tuna and drizzle with the lemon juice-dill mixture. Sprinkle with the remaining 2 tsp. lemon zest and serve with the bulgur salad.

Delicious Chickpea Tuna Salad

INGREDIENTS

2 tablespoons lemon juice

1 tablespoon nonpareil capers, rinsed and chopped

1 tablespoon finely chopped shallot

¼ teaspoon salt

¼ teaspoon ground pepper

1 (15 ounce) can no-salt-added chickpeas, rinsed

1 (6.7 ounce) jar oil-packed tuna, drained

1 cup halved cherry tomatoes

1 cup thinly sliced English cucumber

½ cup crumbled feta cheese

2 tablespoons chopped fresh dill

3 tablespoons extra-virgin olive oil

3 cups baby spinach

INSTRUCTIONS

Stir lemon juice, capers, shallot, salt and pepper together in a large bowl. Let stand for 5 minutes.

Meanwhile, toss chickpeas, tuna, tomatoes, cucumber, feta and dill together in a large bowl.

Whisk oil into the lemon juice mixture until fully incorporated. Spoon about 5 tablespoons of the dressing into the chickpea mixture; toss to coat.

Add spinach to the remaining dressing in the large bowl; toss to coat. Divide the spinach evenly among

4 plates; top each plate with 1 1/4 cups chickpea mixture. Serve immediately.

To make ahead

Prepare through Step 3 and refrigerate in an airtight container for up to 1 day.

Spaghetti Squash with Roasted Tomatoes, Beans & Almond Pesto

INGREDIENTS

Almond Pesto

2 cups fresh basil leaves

1 cup fresh parsley leaves

½ cup grated Parmesan cheese

⅓ cup whole raw almonds

1 clove garlic

1 ½ tablespoons red-wine vinegar

¼ teaspoon kosher salt

¼ teaspoon ground pepper

¼ cup extra-virgin olive oil

¼ cup water

Spaghetti Squash & Vegetables

1 3-pound spaghetti squash

¼ cup water

2 pints grape tomatoes, halved

1 tablespoon extra-virgin olive oil

¼ teaspoon kosher salt

¼ teaspoon ground pepper

1 cup canned cannellini beans, rinsed

INSTRUCTIONS

To prepare pesto: Pulse basil, parsley, Parmesan, almonds, garlic, vinegar and 1/4 teaspoon each salt and pepper in a food processor until coarsely chopped, scraping down the sides. With the motor running, add 1/4 cup oil; process until well combined.

Add water to the pesto in the food processor; pulse to combine.

To prepare squash & vegetables: Preheat oven to 400 degrees F. Line a rimmed baking sheet with foil.

Halve squash lengthwise and scoop out the seeds. Place cut-side down in a microwave-safe dish and add water. Microwave on High until the flesh can be easily scraped with a fork, about 15 minutes.

Meanwhile, toss tomatoes with oil, salt and pepper in a large bowl. Transfer to the prepared baking sheet. Roast until soft and wrinkled, 10 to 12 minutes. Remove from the oven. Add beans and stir to combine.

Scrape the squash flesh into the bowl and divide among 4 plates. Top each portion with some of the tomato-bean mixture and about 3 tablespoons pesto sauce.

Classic Tuna Niçoise Salad

INGREDIENTS

10 ounces baby yellow or red potatoes (about 2 cups), scrubbed

1 cup halved crosswise fresh green beans

3 tablespoons fresh lemon juice

2 tablespoons finely chopped shallot

1 teaspoon Dijon mustard

½ teaspoon salt, divided

½ teaspoon ground pepper, divided

5 tablespoons extra-virgin olive oil, divided

1 tablespoon chopped fresh flat-leaf parsley

1 (8 ounce) fresh tuna steak

8 cups torn green leaf or Bibb lettuce

2 hard-boiled eggs, peeled and halved lengthwise

1 cup halved cherry tomatoes

½ cup pitted Niçoise olives

INSTRUCTIONS

Place a steamer basket in the bottom of a large pot and add water to just below the bottom of the basket. Cover and bring to a boil over high heat. Add potatoes to the basket and reduce heat to medium; cook, covered, until tender, about 15 minutes. (Do not remove pot from heat.) Transfer potatoes to a plate and let cool for about 10 minutes.

Meanwhile, add green beans to the basket; cook over medium heat, covered, until tender-crisp, about 5 minutes. Transfer the beans to the plate with the potatoes. Cut the cooled potatoes in half crosswise.

Whisk lemon juice, shallot, mustard and 1/4 teaspoon each salt and pepper in a medium bowl until smooth. Whisking constantly, gradually drizzle in 4 tablespoons oil. Whisk in parsley until combined.

Pat tuna dry; sprinkle with the remaining 1/4 teaspoon each salt and pepper. Heat the remaining 1 tablespoon oil in a medium nonstick skillet over medium heat. Add the tuna and cook, turning once, until lightly browned, about 2 minutes per side. Transfer to a clean cutting board and let rest for 5 minutes. Slice 1/2-inch thick against the grain.

Arrange lettuce on a platter or 4 plates; top with the sliced tuna, halved potatoes, green beans, eggs, tomatoes and olives. Drizzle evenly with the dressing and serve immediately.

Butternut Squash & Black Bean Enchiladas

INGREDIENTS

3 tablespoons extra-virgin olive oil, divided

3 cups diced peeled butternut squash

2 medium poblano peppers, seeded and chopped

1 medium onion, chopped

1 (14 ounce) can no-salt-added black beans, rinsed

4 tablespoons chopped fresh cilantro, divided, plus more for serving

1 tablespoon ancho chile powder

8 corn tortillas, warmed

1 (10-ounce) can enchilada sauce (see Tip)

½ cup shredded Monterey Jack cheese

2 cups shredded cabbage

1 tablespoon lime juice

INSTRUCTIONS

Preheat oven to 425°F. Lightly coat a 7-by-11-inch baking dish with cooking spray.

Heat 2 tablespoons oil in a large skillet over medium heat. Add squash and cook, covered, stirring occasionally, until tender and lightly browned, 8 to 10 minutes. Add peppers and onion and cook, uncovered, stirring occasionally, until tender, about 5 minutes. Remove from heat and stir in beans, 2 tablespoons cilantro and chile powder. Let cool for 5 minutes.

Place about 1/2 cup of the squash mixture in each tortilla and roll. Place, seam-side down, in the prepared baking dish. Top with enchilada sauce. Sprinkle with cheese and cover with foil. Bake until bubbly, about 15 minutes. Remove foil and bake for another 5 minutes.

Meanwhile, toss cabbage with lime juice, the remaining 1 tablespoon oil and 2 tablespoons cilantro. Serve the enchiladas topped with the slaw and more cilantro, if desired.

Tip:

Store-bought enchilada sauce is a fast and easy way to add a ton of flavor to a dish, but it can be high in sodium, so look for one that has less than 300 milligrams per serving.

Red Lentil Soup with Saffron

INGREDIENTS

3 tablespoons extra-virgin olive oil

2 medium carrots, finely diced

2 stalks celery, finely diced

1 large onion, finely diced

3 cloves garlic, minced

1 tablespoon tomato paste

½ teaspoon ground cumin

¼ teaspoon crushed saffron threads

¼ teaspoon ground turmeric

4 cups low-sodium no-chicken or chicken broth

1 ½ cups water, plus more as needed

1 pound red lentils (2 cups), picked over and rinsed

5 ounces spinach, coarsely chopped

1 teaspoon kosher salt

1 teaspoon ground pepper

Plain yogurt & chopped fresh mint for garnish

INSTRUCTIONS

Heat oil in a large heavy pot over medium heat. Add carrots, celery and onion and cook until starting to soften, 7 to 10 minutes. (Do not brown.) Stir in garlic, tomato paste, cumin, saffron and turmeric and cook for 1 minute.

Add broth, water, lentils, spinach, salt and pepper. Bring to a simmer. Adjust heat to maintain a simmer, cover and cook, stirring as needed to prevent sticking, until the lentils and vegetables are tender, 15 to 20 minutes. Add more water if desired.

Garnish with yogurt and mint, if desired.

Lemon-Herb Salmon with Caponata & Farro

INGREDIENTS

2 cups water

⅔ cup farro

1 medium eggplant, cut into 1 inch cubes

1 red bell pepper, cut into 1-inch pieces

1 summer squash, cut into 1-inch pieces

1 small onion, cut into 1-inch pieces

1 ½ cups cherry tomatoes

3 tablespoons extra-virgin olive oil

¾ teaspoon salt, divided

½ teaspoon ground pepper, divided

2 tablespoons capers, rinsed and chopped

1 tablespoon red-wine vinegar

2 teaspoons honey

1 ¼ pounds wild salmon (see Tips), cut into 4 portions

1 teaspoon lemon zest

½ teaspoon Italian seasoning

Lemon wedges for serving

INSTRUCTIONS

Position racks in upper and lower thirds of oven; preheat to 450 degrees F. Line 2 rimmed baking sheets with foil and coat with cooking spray.

Bring water and farro to a boil in a saucepan. Reduce heat to low, cover and simmer until just tender, about 30 minutes. Drain if necessary.

Meanwhile, toss eggplant, bell pepper, squash, onion and tomatoes with oil, 1/2 teaspoon salt and 1/4 teaspoon pepper in a large bowl. Divide between the prepared baking sheets. Roast on the upper and lower racks, stirring once halfway, until the vegetables are tender and starting to brown, about 25 minutes. Return them to the bowl. Stir in capers, vinegar and honey.

Season salmon with lemon zest, Italian seasoning and the remaining 1/4 teaspoon each salt and pepper and place on one of the baking sheets. Roast on the lower rack until just cooked through, 6 to 12 minutes, depending on thickness. Serve the salmon with the farro, vegetable caponata and lemon wedges.

Tomatoes with Garlic & Olives

INGREDIENTS

1 pint cherry tomatoes, halved

¼ cup Kalamata olives, quartered

2 tablespoons extra-virgin olive oil, divided

4 teaspoons minced garlic

1 tablespoon chopped fresh thyme

½ teaspoon salt, divided

½ teaspoon ground pepper, divided

1 ¼ pounds salmon fillet, cut into 4 portions

INSTRUCTIONS

Preheat oven to 400 degrees F.

Stir tomatoes, olives, 1 tablespoon oil, garlic, thyme, 1/4 teaspoon salt and 1/4 teaspoon pepper together in a medium bowl. Spread the mixture on half of a large rimmed sheet pan. Brush the remaining 1 tablespoon oil all over the salmon pieces; sprinkle with the remaining 1/4 teaspoon each salt and pepper. Place on the empty side of the sheet pan. Bake until the tomatoes have broken down and the salmon is just cooked through, 12 to 15 minutes. Serve the tomato mixture atop the salmon.

White Bean Soup with Pasta

INGREDIENTS

1 tablespoon extra-virgin olive oil

1 ½ cups frozen mirepoix (diced onion, celery and carrot)

2 cloves garlic, minced

1 teaspoon Italian seasoning

1 teaspoon salt

¼ teaspoon crushed red pepper

¼ teaspoon ground pepper

1 28-ounce can no-salt-added diced tomatoes

2 cups low-sodium no-chicken broth or chicken broth

1 15-ounce can low-sodium cannellini beans, rinsed

8 ounces small whole-wheat pasta, such as elbows

1 ½ cups frozen cut-leaf spinach

4 tablespoons grated Parmesan cheese

INSTRUCTIONS

Put a large saucepan of water on to boil.

Heat oil in a large pot over medium-high heat. Add mirepoix and cook, stirring, until softened, about 3 minutes. Add garlic, Italian seasoning, salt, crushed red pepper and ground pepper and cook, stirring, until fragrant, about 1 minute. Add tomatoes and their juices, broth and beans and bring to a boil. Reduce heat to maintain a lively simmer. Cover and cook, stirring occasionally, until the tomatoes begin to break down, about 10 minutes.

Meanwhile, cook pasta in the boiling water for 1 minute less than the package directions. Drain.

Stir spinach into the soup. Stir in the pasta just before serving. Serve topped with Parmesan.

Spanish Omelette

INGREDIENTS

450g potatoes peeled and sliced

1 teaspoon olive oil

1 red onion, diced

½ red pepper, de-seeded and diced

1 tablespoon fresh parsley, chopped

4 large eggs

½ tbsp grated Parmesan

Black pepper

INSTRUCTIONS

Cook the potato slices in a pan of boiling water until tender (about 5 minutes).

Meanwhile, cook the onion and pepper in a frying pan with the oil until softened.

Add the potatoes and gently combine.

Beat the eggs in a bowl, add the parsley, parmesan and black pepper and mix thoroughly.

Pour into the frying pan and allow the bottom of the egg mixture to set – about 3 minutes.

Finish by cooking under a hot grill taking care not to burn the omelette - another 3 minutes.

Serve with a sliced tomato salad.

Lentil Stew with Salsa Verde

INGREDIENTS

1 tablespoon olive oil

1 ¼ cups finely chopped celery (4-6 stalks) or fennel (1 bulb)

3 small carrots, peeled and finely chopped (1/2 cup)

½ cup finely chopped red bell pepper

5 tablespoons finely chopped shallot (1 large), divided

2 large cloves garlic, minced

2 tablespoons tomato paste

1 ½ cups French green lentils, sorted and rinsed

4 cups low-sodium chicken broth or vegetable broth, or water

¾ teaspoon ground pepper, divided

½ teaspoon salt, divided

1 small bunch Italian parsley, finely chopped (about 3/4 cup)

1 large lime, juiced (2 Tbsp.)

2 tablespoons white-wine vinegar

INSTRUCTIONS

Heat oil in a 4- to 6-qt. pot over medium-high heat. Add celery (or fennel), carrots, bell pepper, 3 Tbsp. shallot, and garlic. Cook, stirring, until softened, about 3 minutes. Add tomato paste; cook, stirring, for 30 seconds. Add lentils, broth (or water), 1/2 tsp. pepper, and 1/4 tsp. salt. Bring to a boil. Cover, reduce heat to low, and simmer until the lentils are tender, 35 to 40 minutes.

Meanwhile, combine parsley, lime juice, vinegar, and the remaining 2 Tbsp. shallot and 1/4 tsp. each pepper and salt in a small bowl; stir well.

To serve, divide the stew among 4 bowls and top each with a dollop of the salsa verde. Pass the remaining salsa verde separately.

To make ahead

Prepare stew through Step 1. Refrigerate for up to 3 days. Reheat on the stovetop or in the microwave, adding water if necessary.

Black Bean Wraps with Greens

INGREDIENTS

1 cup chopped fresh cilantro

3 tablespoons white-wine vinegar

2 cloves garlic, peeled

1 teaspoon ground cumin, divided

½ teaspoon salt, divided

¼ cup extra-virgin olive oil

3 cups chopped romaine lettuce

1 cup chopped radicchio

1 cup sliced radishes

1 (15 ounce) can no-salt-added black beans, rinsed

½ teaspoon chili powder

½ teaspoon garlic powder

1 ripe avocado

1 tablespoon lime juice

4 (8 inch) whole-wheat tortillas or wraps

INSTRUCTIONS

Combine cilantro, vinegar, garlic, 1/2 teaspoon cumin and 1/4 teaspoon salt in a mini food processor; pulse until finely chopped. With the motor running, slowly stream in oil. Transfer the vinaigrette to a large bowl. Add lettuce, radicchio and radishes and toss to coat.

Mash beans, chili powder, garlic powder, the remaining 1/2 teaspoon cumin and 1/4 teaspoon salt in a medium bowl. Mash avocado with lime juice in a small bowl. Spread some of the mashed beans and avocado over each tortilla; top with the salad and roll up.

Chopped Veggie Grain Bowls with Turmeric Dressing

INGREDIENTS

2 (8 ounce) packages cooked quinoa

1 (16 ounce) container chopped veggie mix

1 (15.5 ounce) can chickpeas, rinsed

1/2 cup creamy turmeric salad dressing

INSTRUCTIONS

Prepare quinoa according to package directions. Transfer to a shallow bowl to cool completely before assembling bowls.

Divide veggie mix among 4 single-serving lidded containers. Top each with one-fourth of the quinoa and one-fourth of the chickpeas. Seal the containers and refrigerate for up to 4 days.

Transfer 2 tablespoons salad dressing into each of 4 small lidded containers and refrigerate for up to 4 days.

Toss each bowl with dressing just before serving.

CHAPTER VIII

GALLSTONE-FRIENDLY APPETIZER RECIPES FOR SENIORS

Homemade Salsa

INGREDIENTS

2 cups chopped tomatoes

¼ cup chopped red onion

¼ cup chopped yellow onion

2 tablespoons canned green chilies

2 tablespoons fresh lime juice

2 tablespoons chopped fresh cilantro

2 cloves garlic, peeled

1 teaspoon ground cumin

¼ teaspoon salt

INSTRUCTIONS

Gather all ingredients.

Combine tomatoes, red onion, yellow onion, green chilies, lime juice, cilantro, garlic, cumin, and salt in a food processor.

Pulse until mixture is combined but still chunky.

Transfer salsa to a bowl, cover with plastic wrap, and refrigerate at least 1 hour before serving.

Serve with chips.

Tomatillo Salsa Verde

INGREDIENTS

1 pound tomatillos, husked

½ cup finely chopped onion

1 serrano chile pepper, minced

1 teaspoon minced garlic

2 tablespoons chopped cilantro

1 tablespoon chopped fresh oregano

1 ½ teaspoons salt, or to taste

½ teaspoon ground cumin

2 cups water

INSTRUCTIONS

Gather all ingredients.

Place tomatillos, onion, chile pepper, and garlic into a large saucepan; season with cilantro, oregano, salt, and cumin. Pour in water and bring to a boil over high heat; reduce heat to medium-low and simmer until the tomatillos are soft, 10 to 15 minutes.

Transfer tomatillo mixture into a blender in batches; puree until smooth. If you prefer a thicker salsa verde, use a slotted spoon to transfer the tomatillo mixture into a blender, then add cooking water as needed to reach the desired consistency.

Serve with chips.

Puerto Rican Tostones

INGREDIENTS

1 green plantain

5 tablespoons oil for frying

3 cups cold water

salt to taste

INSTRUCTIONS

Peel plantain and cut into 1-inch slices. Fill a bowl with 3 cups of cold water.

Heat oil in a large deep skillet over medium-high heat; add plantain slices in an even layer and fry on both sides until golden brown, about 3 1/2 minutes per side. Set skillet aside.

Transfer plantain slices to a chopping board; flatten each one by placing a small plate on top and pressing down. Dip plantain slices in cold water.

Reheat oil in the skillet over medium heat; cook plantain slices for 1 minute on each side. Season to taste with salt and serve immediately.

Classic Chili Lime Crispy Chickpeas

INGREDIENTS

for 4 servings

15.5 oz chickpeas(440 g), 1 can, drained and rinsed

2 teaspoons olive oil

1 teaspoon chili powder

¾ teaspoon salt

¼ teaspoon black pepper

1 lime, zested

1 lime, juiced

INSTRUCTIONS

Preheat oven to 350°F (180°C).

In a bowl, toss the chickpeas with olive oil, chili powder, salt, pepper, lime zest, and lime juice.

Transfer chickpeas to a parchment paper-lined baking sheet and bake for 35 minutes, until crispy.

Enjoy!

INSTRUCTIONS

Preheat oven to 350°F (180°C).

In a bowl, toss the chickpeas with olive oil, chili powder, salt, pepper, lime zest, and lime juice.

Transfer chickpeas to a parchment paper-lined baking sheet and bake for 35 minutes, until crispy.

Enjoy!

Sriracha Buffalo Cauliflower Bites

INGREDIENTS

for 2 servings

1 large head cauliflower

½ cup flour(70 g)

1 teaspoon garlic powder

¾ cup unsweetened almond milk(180 mL)

⅓ cup sriracha sauce(105 g)

⅓ cup buffalo sauce(110 g)

INSTRUCTIONS

Preheat oven to 400°F (200°C).

Break the head of cauliflower into bite-sized florets.

In a large bowl, combine flour, garlic powder, almond milk and Sriracha.

Add the cauliflower florets and coat well.

Transfer the coated florets onto a parchment-lined baking sheet and bake for 20 minutes.

Remove the cauliflower from the oven and allow to cool for a few minutes.

Once cool, transfer into a bowl, add buffalo sauce and coat well.

Return cauliflower to the baking sheet and bake for 10 more minutes or until heated through.

Serve with ranch or your favorite dipping sauce.

Savory Crispy Chicken Strips And Veggies

INGREDIENTS

for 4 servings

CRISPY CHICKEN STRIPS

4 boneless, skinless chicken breasts

2 large eggs

3 tablespoons extra virgin olive oil, divided

1 ½ cups panko breadcrumbs(75 g)

2 teaspoons paprika

1 ½ teaspoons kosher salt, divided

1 cup all-purpose flour(125 g)

2 cups broccoli florets(300 g)

½ teaspoon ground black pepper, divided

2 cloves garlic, minced, divided

2 sweet potatoes, peeled

DIPPING SAUCE

½ cup mayonnaise(120 g)

2 tablespoons dijon mustard

2 teaspoons honey

BBQ sauce, for serving, optional

ketchup, for serving, optional

INSTRUCTIONS

Preheat the oven to 375°F (190°C) and line 2 baking sheets with parchment paper.

Slice the chicken breasts into strips.

In a medium bowl, whisk together the eggs and 1 tablespoon of olive oil.

In a large bowl, combine the panko bread crumbs, paprika, and 1 teaspoon of salt.

Place the flour in another medium bowl.

Coat the chicken strips in the flour, then in the eggs, then in the bread crumbs, and place on a baking sheet.

In a large bowl, toss the broccoli florets with the 1 tablespoon olive oil, ¼ teaspoon salt, ¼ teaspoon pepper, and half of the minced garlic. Arrange on half of the remaining baking sheet.

Cut the sweet potatoes in half lengthwise, then slice into half-moons.

Toss the sweet potatoes in a large bowl with the remaining tablespoon of olive oil, ¼ teaspoon salt,

¼ teaspoon pepper, and minced garlic, and place on the baking sheet next to the broccoli.

Bake both baking sheets simultaneously, until the veggies are browned and the chicken is crisp, about 20 minutes.

Make the dipping sauce: Combine the mayonnaise, mustard, and honey in a small bowl.

Serve the chicken and veggies with the dipping sauce, BBQ sauce, and ketchup, if using.

Summer Cauliflower Salad

INGREDIENTS

for 4 servings

1 head cauliflower, cut into florets

olive oil

kosher salt

freshly ground black pepper

3 hard-boiled eggs, peeled

6 slices bacon, cooked

¼ cup shredded cheddar cheese (25 g)

2 scallions, thinly sliced, plus more for garnish

DRESSING

1 tablespoon French's yellow mustard

⅔ cup mayonnaise (160 g)

2 tablespoons lemon juice

½ teaspoon garlic powder

¼ teaspoon paprika

½ teaspoon freshly ground black pepper

1 teaspoon kosher salt

INSTRUCTIONS

Preheat oven to 400ºF.

In a bowl, toss cauliflower with olive oil, salt, and pepper. Spread in an even layer on a parchment-lined baking sheet. Roast for 20–25 minutes, stirring halfway through, until edges of the cauliflower start to brown and florets are tender. Remove from oven, let cool for a few minutes, then transfer to a large bowl.

Slice hard-boiled eggs in half, then slice each half into 4 pieces. Roughly chop the bacon slices. Add the eggs and bacon to the bowl, along with cheddar cheese and scallions.

In a separate bowl, whisk dressing ingredients together until smooth. Pour dressing over cauliflower and toss to coat everything well. Garnish with extra sliced scallions before serving.

CHAPTER IX

GALLSTONE-FRIENDLY SALAD RECIPES FOR SENIORS

Pesto Pasta Salad

INGREDIENTS

Pea pesto

200g frozen peas

20g pine nuts

A handful fresh basil

1½ tsp olive oil

The juice of one lemon

Pepper to taste

The pasta

1 tsp olive oil

350g Quorn Pieces

65g kale

400g cooked wholewheat pasta

65g baby spinach

3 spring onions, sliced

Fresh thyme, finely chopped

INSTRUCTIONS

Pea Pesto

Thaw the peas overnight in the fridge, or place in a bowl and cover with freshly boiled water and leave for 5 minutes before draining.

Place the peas, pine nuts, basil, and olive oil in a food processor and blend until smooth. Add the lemon juice and pepper to taste.

The Pasta

Heat 1 tsp of olive oil in a pan, add the Quorn Pieces and fry until golden. Add the kale and fry for 3 more minutes.

Place the cooked pasta into a bowl and add the Quorn kale mixture, spinach, onions, thyme and pea pesto and mix well.

Each serving of this recipe provides 23g of protein** and 15g of fibre*. The UK government recommends that adults should consume 30g of fibre daily.

Picnic Salad with Vegetarian Chicken Style Pieces

INGREDIENTS

3 heaped tbsp sweetcorn kernels, canned or frozen

200g Quorn Pieces

200g dry pasta, cooked to manufacturer's instructions

250g cherry tomatoes, rinsed and halved

50g bean sprouts

1 bag of lettuce leaves, rinsed

1 400g can of black beans, drained and rinsed

1 can of chickpeas, drained and rinsed

1 tsp rapeseed (vegetable) oil

50g toasted sunflower seeds

A few pickled jalapeños, sliced, for serving (optional)

Marinade:

25ml Alpro soya drink or other plant-based drinks

25ml rapeseed oil

2 tablespoons honey

1 squeezed lime

INSTRUCTIONS

If using frozen sweetcorn, remove from the freezer and allow to thaw in the fridge overnight. If using canned, drain and rinse.

Mix the ingredients for the marinade and pour it into a bag of frozen Quorn Pieces, let the bag stand to marinate.

Boil the pasta according to the instructions on the package.

Mix the cooked pasta, sweetcorn, chickpeas, black beans, tomatoes, bean sprouts and lettuce leaves.

Fry the Quorn Pieces on medium heat with a teaspoon of oil to warm through.

Top the salad with the Quorn Pieces, toasted sunflower seeds and, if using, pickled jalapeños.

*This recipe is a source of protein. Each serving provides 27g of protein.

Winter California Walnut Slaw

INGREDIENTS

100g California Walnut pieces

400g red cabbage, finely shredded

1 fennel bulb, approx. 300g, finely shredded

1 medium eating apple, cored and coarsely grated

1 small red onion, finely sliced

25g parsley, chopped

100g reduced fat mayonnaise

50g creamed horseradish

2 tbsp cider vinegar

INSTRUCTIONS

Preheat the oven to 200C, gas mark 6.

Place the walnuts in a small roasting tin and roast for 6-8 minutes, set aside to cool.

Meanwhile, mix together the cabbage, fennel, apple, onion and parsley in a large bowl.

In a separate bowl, mix together the mayonnaise, horseradish and vinegar, season well and stir into the slaw. Stir in the walnuts, reserving a few to scatter over the top.

Super Christmas Salad

INGREDIENTS

450g sweet potato, diced

2 tbsp olive oil

¼ ciabatta loaf, torn into bite sized pieces

50g Walnut Halves

150g kale

200g cooked roast turkey, torn into pieces

50g pomegranate seeds

3-4 tbsp reduced fat Caesar dressing

INSTRUCTIONS

Preheat the oven to 200oC, gas mark 6.

Place the sweet potatoes on a baking tray and toss in 1 tbsp oil then roast for 20 minutes or until tender. Remove to a bowl to cool. Add the ciabatta to the same tray and toss in the remaining oil, cook for 5 minutes then scatter the walnuts to one side of the tray and roast for a further 5-8 minutes until golden.

Meanwhile, cook the kale in boiling water for 2-3 minutes, drain and run under cold water, squeeze out excess liquid.

Toss kale with the sweet potato, turkey and pomegranate seeds and place on a serving platter. Top with the ciabatta croutons and walnuts, drizzle over the dressing and serve.

Loch Duart Salmon Nicoise with Charred Lemon Dressing

INGREDIENTS

200g Baby Potatoes

1.5 tablespoons of Rapeseed Oil

500g Loch Duart Salmon Fillet

100g Green Beans

3 Eggs, medium size

2 Lemons, halved

1 clove of Garlic, minced

100g Cherry tomatoes, halved

50g Black Olives

Half a Cucumber, cut into chunks

50g of radishes, quartered

Handful of mixed leaves

Black pepper

INSTRUCTIONS

Preheat the oven to 200 degrees.

Cut the baby potatoes in half and coat them with a small drizzle of oil and season with pepper. When the oven is hot, roast them on a tray for 15-20 minutes, turning halfway through.

Whilst the potatoes are roasting, get on prepping the rest of the ingredients. Bring a small pot of water to a boil and slowly lower the eggs in. Set a timer for 6 minutes. If the eggs have been in the fridge, increase the cooking time by 1 minute. When done, run under cold water, peel and set aside in the water to cool completely.

Heat a non-stick frying pan over a medium heat. Once hot, brush the lemon with a little oil to prevent sticking and place them cut side down. Don't be tempted to move them around too much. Cook until the lemons are heated through and charred on the cut side, about 3 minutes.

Once the potatoes are done, remove from the oven and set aside.

Turn the oven down to 180 degrees. Place the salmon on an oven tray and brush over a small amount of rapeseed oil, season with pepper. Place into the oven and roast for 20 minutes. When the salmon has had 10 minutes of cooking time, add the green beans to the oven tray and continue to roast for the remaining time.

To make the dressing whisk together a tablespoon of rapeseed oil with the minced garlic clove, juice from a half of the grilled lemon, and a pinch of pepper.

Scatter the mixed leaves on a platter and arrange the other ingredients in sections. Tear the eggs into halves and season. Break the warm salmon into large pieces and place onto the platter. Drizzle the salad with the dressing and serve.

Salmon with Potato Salad and Horseradish Yogurt

INGREDIENTS

600g baby potatoes

4 skin-on Loch Duart Salmon fillets

2 tbsp of vegetable oil (for frying the salmon)

¾ tsp of caraway seeds, coarsely chopped

Potato Dressing

50ml of vegetable oil

1 tbsp of white wine vinegar

2 tbsp of freshly chopped dill

Freshly ground black pepper

Horseradish Yoghurt

1 tbsp horseradish sauce

1 tsp white wine vinegar

250ml 0% fat Greek yogurt

1 tbsp of olive oil

Freshly ground black pepper

INSTRUCTIONS

Place potatoes in a medium pot. Pour in water to cover and bring to a boil; reduce heat and gently simmer until tender, 20–25 minutes.

For the dressing, whisk 50ml of vegetable oil and 1 tbsp of white wine vinegar in a bowl big enough to hold the potatoes. Whisk half of the dill into the dressing, season with pepper. Set remaining dill aside for serving.

In a small bowl combine the horseradish, 1 tsp of white wine vinegar, and season with a pinch of salt if necessary; let it sit for 5 minutes. Whisk in yogurt and 1 tbsp of olive oil. Season with pepper.

Preheat a frying pan over a medium heat. Rub both sides of the salmon fillets with the vegetable oil and season with salt and pepper. Place skin side down in the pan and cook until skin is crispy, 6-8 minutes. Turn the fish over and turn off the heat. Add the caraway seeds and allow the fish to cook through in the residual heat of the pan.

As soon as the potatoes are done cooking, drain and add to bowl with dressing. Toss to coat and season with more pepper if needed.

To serve, place a spoonful of horseradish yogurt onto each plate, top with salmon fillet and serve potatoes alongside. Sprinkle with the rest of the dill.

Coleslaw - 100% plant-based!

INGREDIENTS

1 small white cabbage, finely shredded

3 carrots, grated

1 red apple, cored and sliced

3 spring onions, finely sliced

60g unsalted cashew nuts or peanuts

1 tbsp sesame seeds

Dressing

200g Alpro Plain Soya alternative to Greek Style Yogurt

1 tbsp white wine vinegar

1 tbsp maple/agave syrup

1 tbsp lemon juice

2 tsp Dijon mustard

INSTRUCTIONS

Prep the veggies. Finely chop the cabbage and coarsely grate the carrot. Slice the apple and spring onions. Then pop the whole lot into a large bowl and toss together.

Now for the dressing. Mix the Alpro Plain soya alternative to Greek Style yogurt, vinegar, agave syrup, lemon juice and mustard and season with a pinch of salt and pepper. Mix together until smooth and creamy.

Pour the dressing over the salad mix and stir through until all the veggies are nicely coated.

Finally, for a little extra crunch, coarsely chop the nuts and scatter over the salad along with the sesame seeds. The perfect side for summer BBQs.

Dukkah-crusted halloumi salad

INGREDIENTS

100g lettuce, shredded

1 large spring onion, thinly sliced

2 tomatoes, chopped

1/8 cucumber, chopped

70g cooked beetroot, chopped

4 radishes, sliced

75g light halloumi cheese, chopped into 2cm cubes

2 tsp Dukkah

For the dressing

2 level tbsp mango chutney

½ tsp white wine vinegar

6 drops of Tabasco sauce

INSTRUCTIONS

Pre-heat the grill. Line a grill pan with foil.

Divide the lettuce, spring onion, tomatoes, cucumber, beetroot and radishes between two plates.

Mix together the chopped halloumi and Dukkah in a bowl.

Transfer the coated halloumi and any excess Dukkah into the grill pan. Cook under the grill for a couple of minutes, turning once, until the Dukkah is lightly toasted.

Remove and add to the salad vegetables.

Heat a small saucepan over a medium heat, quickly add the mango chutney, white wine vinegar, tabasco and 40mls of water. Bubble for 20 to 30 seconds. You may need a little more vinegar depending on which brand of mango chutney you use. Pour the dressing over the salad and eat immediately.

Mackerel with Red Pepper Quinoa Salad

INGREDIENTS

4 fresh mackerel fillets

200g quinoa

1.5 litres of good quality low-salt vegetable stock

80g rocket

2 cloves of garlic

1 red chilli

170g sugar snap peas or mangetout

250g red pepper, roasted (and rinsed if from a jar)

1 tbsp olive oil

1 small red onion

To serve, young salad leaves

INSTRUCTIONS

For the quinoa salad, put the quinoa into a saucepan with 400ml of the vegetable stock. Bring to the boil and then let simmer for 10 minutes before removing from the heat. Allow the quinoa to absorb any remaining stock.

Meanwhile, add the rocket, garlic, chilli and 100ml of the vegetable stock to a food processor and blend until smooth.

Bring the remaining stock to the boil, add the sugar snap peas/mangetout and boil for 3-5 minutes.

For the mackerel, heat the olive oil in a frying pan. Add the mackerel and fry for 2 minutes on each side and then remove from the pan.

Once the peas/mange tout are cooked, add them to the quinoa, diced red onion, rocket mixture and roasted red peppers. Mix well and serve with the mackerel. Scatter over the young salad leaves if using

Tuna Beetroot Avocado and Walnut Salad

INGREDIENTS

3 ripe avocados

6 (480g) whole beetroots, cooked & ready to eat (not in vinegar)

3 small tins of tuna in water, about 210g tuna meat

3 clementines, segmented

120g walnuts/walnut pieces

3 tbsp extra virgin olive oil

6 tbsp good quality balsamic vinegar

Handful of basil leaves

INSTRUCTIONS

Peel and slice the avocados, slice the beetroots and display them around the plate or salad bowl.

Roughly chop the walnuts and sprinkle these over the avocado and beets along with the tuna and Clementine segments.

In a jug, whisk together the olive oil and balsamic vinegar and drizzle over the salad. Finish by decorating the top with some basil leaves.

Mango salad with Quorn Fillets

INGREDIENTS

1 pack frozen Quorn Vegetarian Fillets

Splash of oil, for frying

250g pack cherry tomatoes, halved

Small handful coriander, roughly chopped

Zest & juice of 1 lime, plus wedges to serve

1 small red onion, finely sliced

2 garlic cloves, crushed

1 tbsp olive oil

2 little gem lettuce, torn into bite-sized pieces

1 red pepper, deseeded and finely sliced

1 ripe mango (~230g), peeled, stoned and flesh diced

Small handful (15g) tortilla chips, broken up a little

INSTRUCTIONS

Defrost the Quorn Fillets overnight in the fridge. Once thawed, slice into strips and fry over medium heat, with a drizzle of oil until lightly golden. Remove and set aside until needed.

Place the cherry tomatoes, coriander, lime juice and zest, onion, garlic and oil in a large bowl and mix well.

Add the pan-fried strips of Quorn Fillets, lettuce, red pepper and mango. Mix to coat.

Sprinkle the tortilla chips over the top and serve immediately with lime wedges.

CHEFS TIP: No little gem lettuce in the house? No problem! You could use baby spinach, kale or rocket instead.

BBQ Teriyaki Fillets and Pineapple Buddha Bowl

INGREDIENTS

For the skewers:

Half a pack (150-160g) of Quorn Fillets, defrosted

2 thick slices (~350g) fresh or 4-5 canned pineapple slices in juice, drained

For the teriyaki marinade:

150ml water

2 tsp of reduced salt soy sauce

2 tsp sesame oil

1 tbsp mirin

½ tbsp maple syrup

½ tbsp arrowroot powder

1 clove of garlic, minced

1 tbsp fresh ginger, grated

¼ tsp black pepper

For the salad:

1 pack (~250g) of pre-cooked quinoa

80g romaine lettuce, shredded

50g red cabbage, shredded

½ red pepper, finely sliced

1 carrot, grated

2 spring onions, finely sliced

80g ready-to-eat edamame beans

1/2 cucumber, sliced into ribbons

4 radishes, finely sliced

Garnishes:

5g fresh coriander, finely chopped

1 red chilli, finely chopped

1 tbsp toasted sesame seeds

1 tbsp peanuts, crushed

4 wedges of lime

INSTRUCTIONS

If using wooden skewers, soak them in water (fully submerge) for at least 30 minutes before using.

Place the whole Quorn Fillets and pineapple slices onto skewers (soaked if wooden) and set aside.

Make the Teriyaki marinade: put all the ingredients into a small pan and set over a medium heat, whisking constantly until the sauce thickens. Set ¼ of the sauce to one side. Using a pastry brush, coat the skewered Quorn and pineapple pieces with the remaining ¾ of the sauce.

Place the skewers onto a pre-heated gas or charcoal BBQ and cook for 12-15 minutes, turning them occasionally.

Whilst the fillets and pineapple are cooking, make the salad: take a large bowl and mix together the quinoa, lettuce, red cabbage, red pepper, carrot, and spring onions.

Once cooked, remove the fillets and pineapple from the skewers. Slice the fillets diagonally and roughly chop the pineapple and place them to the side.

Divide the salad between four bowls and place fillets and pineapple pieces, edamame beans, cucumber ribbons and radishes on top of the salad.

Garnish with coriander, red chilli, sesame seeds and crushed peanuts. Drizzle with the remaining teriyaki sauce and serve with the lime wedges.

*Provides 15g of protein per serving

CHAPTER X
THE ROLE OF NUTRITION IN PREVENTION AND MANAGEMENT OF GALLSTONE

Nutrition is pivotal in both preventing and managing gallstones. Certain dietary habits can significantly lower the risk of developing symptomatic gallstone disease. For instance, the Mediterranean and DASH (Dietary Approaches to Stop Hypertension) diets have been shown to reduce the risk of gallstone disease. These diets emphasize lean proteins, whole foods, and healthy fats while limiting added sugars, processed foods, and unhealthy fats.

www.ingramcontent.com/pod-product-compliance
Lightning Source LLC
Chambersburg PA
CBHW071830210526
45479CB00001B/63